Delicious Fruit Infused Water For Weight Loss

25 recipes for Spa Quality Fruit Infused water to Supercharge Weight Loss

By: Janice Janoski

Table of Contents

An Intro To Fruit Water And Its Many Benefits — 3

What You Need To Get Started — 4

The Basic Gist Of Making Fruit Waters — 5

Day Spa Inspired Recipes — 6
- Red Dream Fruit Water — 6
- The Weight Loss Water — 7
- The Rejuvenator — 7
- The Herbalist — 8
- Lemon-Lavender Water — 9
- The Spa Lunch — 9
- The Ginger Mint Snap — 10
- The Lover's Lane — 11

Our Favorite Fruit Water Recipes For Summer — 12
- The Summer Stand — 12
- The Red, Light, And Blue — 12
- The Chillo — 13
- The Mini Mojito — 14
- The Sugar-Sugar — 14
- The Strawberry Smash Hit — 15
- The Egyptian Classic — 16
- The Apple Pie — 16
- The Pucker Delight — 17

Tea Infused Fruit Waters — 18
- The Raspberry Green Tea Special — 18
- Old School Lemon Tea — 18

The Just Plain Tasty — 19
- The Melon-Basil Twist — 19
- The Blackberry-Orange Mixer — 20
- The Green Machine — 20

The Apple Ginger Kicker   *21*
Feeling Blue?   *22*
The Cherry Pie   *22*

Enjoy This Book?   **23**

An Intro To Fruit Water And Its Many Benefits

Weight loss and good health always are linked to avid consumption of one important drink – water. The problem with water is that, for many people, it gets really old, really fast. Plain water is not like soda. It has no flavor, no zing, no pizazz to speak of that could give it an extra refreshing boost. So, dieters that are addicted to flavor have a tendency of getting less water in their diet than they should. The solution to this dilemma is simple. Instead of sodas and other unhealthy beverages, it's better to drink water that's been infused with fruit flavoring using natural methods.

There are many, many perks to having a diet that involves fruit infused water instead of diet soda. The most obvious one is that diet soda does still have a lot of chemicals in it that don't exactly make it the healthiest thing in the world to ingest. Water, on the other hand, improves skin tone, boosts your metabolism, and also helps flush out toxins. Soda – even the calorie-free kind – has been, on the other hand, linked to weight gain and attention span disorders in children. Fruit water, unlike sodas, often has antioxidants and vitamins from the fruit and herbs

I sincerely hope that you did!

As a self-publisher, reviews do so much to help grow the audience for this book.

Would you do me the honor of leaving a review and let me know what you think?

Even one small sentence would be so wonderful!

Thank you so much!

Janice

3. Place the pitcher in the fridge for 24 hours. Strain the solids out of the water using cheesecloth or a fine strainer.
4. Serve chilled, with an equally colorful meal!

The Cherry Pie

It's really hard not to love the deliciously sweet taste of black cherries. This recipe highlights how awesome cherries can be, and how easily they can turn regular water into an amazing thirst quenching beverage.

Ingredients:

- 10 black cherries, halved and pitted
- 4 strawberries, sliced
- Ice and water

How To Make It:

1. Place the cherries and strawberries at the bottom of a pitcher.
2. Fill the rest of the pitcher with ice and water. Stir.
3. Let the mixture sit in a fridge for approximately 24 hours.
4. Serve chilled.

Enjoy This Book?

How To Make It:

1. Place the ginger, vanilla bean, apple slices, and lemon slice into a pitcher.
2. Fill up the rest of the pitcher with ice water. Place the pitcher into the fridge and leave it overnight.
3. Remove the solids using a strainer. Toss the apple slices back in, and serve. Add honey to taste.

Feeling Blue?

Sometimes, we just get the urge to eat or drink something really colorful. Nothing is more colorful or more eye-catching than this beautifully blue drink!

Ingredients:

- ½ cup blueberries
- ½ cup blackberries
- ½ cup red grapes
- ½ cup black currant
- Ice and water

How To Make It:

1. Using a spoon, crush all the berries and fruits in a small bowl. Place the resulting mixture into a pitcher.
2. Fill the pitcher up with ice water. Stir for about 1 minute.

Ingredients:

- 6 Granny Smith apple slices
- ½ starfruit, sliced thinly
- ¼ lime, sliced thinly
- ½ kiwi, sliced thinly
- Ice and Water

How To Make It:

1. Add all the fruit to the pitcher.
2. Fill the remaining pitcher space with water and ice.
3. Place the pitcher in the fridge, and leave it for 12 to 24 hours.
4. Serve, garnishing the drink with an extra star fruit slice.

The Apple Ginger Kicker

If you love the flavor of apples, and want to experience a unique kick to it, this is your new go-to drink. Trust us when we say that this gets very spicy, very quickly!

Ingredients:

- Water and ice
- 10 slices Gala apples
- 1 tablespoon sliced ginger
- 1 vanilla bean
- 1 slice lemon
- Honey (optional)

How To Make It:

1. Place the basil, rosemary, watermelon and blackberries in a pitcher.
2. Add the water and ice to the fill line.
3. Place the pitcher in the fridge, and wait 24 hours for it to steep.
4. Remove the basil and rosemary, and serve chilled.

The Blackberry-Orange Mixer

Blackberries are a great ingredient in any fruit water combination. In this case, the natural sugary sweetness of blackberries is compounded by the tart yet sweet taste of orange. Yummy!

Ingredients:

- 1 handful of blackberries
- ¼ orange, thinly sliced
- Ice and water

How To Make It:

1. Place the blackberries and orange slices in the pitcher. Fill up the rest of the pitcher with ice water.
2. Place in the fridge for 12 to 18 hours.
3. Strain the infusion, and serve.

The Green Machine

What do you get when you mix green apples, star fruit, lime, kiwi, and water? You end up with a thirst quencher unlike anything else you've ever tasted!

Ingredients:

- 1 pitcher of pre-prepared black tea
- ½ lemon, sliced thinly
- Honey (optional)

How To Make It:

1. Add the lemon to the pitcher of black tea.
2. Let it sit in the fridge overnight.
3. Serve with breakfast, lunch or dinner. Add honey to taste.

The Just Plain Tasty

These aren't recipes that we can include in any particular category. However, we still find them to be amazing in taste, and healthy as can be. They are just downright tasty!

The Melon-Basil Twist

For people who enjoy the taste of watermelon, and the refreshing herbal taste of basil, this recipe is just what the doctor ordered.

Ingredients:

- 4 small slices of watermelon, chopped up into tiny pieces
- 1 handful of basil
- 1 sprig of rosemary
- 1 handful of blackberries
- Ice and water

Tea Infused Fruit Waters

Nothing is better than sipping on hot tea…unless it's sipping on an amazing blend of tea and fruit! Here are some amazing recipes for the tea lover in all of us.

The Raspberry Green Tea Special

This wonderful recipe involves the weight-loss inducing power of green tea with the tart yet tasty flavor of raspberry. What's there not to love?

Ingredients:

- 1 packet macha green tea powder, unsweetened
- 1 handful of raspberries
- Water and ice

How To Make It:

1. Use a spoon to gently press on the raspberries until juice leaks out. Drop the raspberries into the pitcher.
2. Add the green tea powder and ice water. Stir until the green tea has been thoroughly mixed in.
3. Place the pitcher in a fridge for 12 hours, and then serve.

Old School Lemon Tea

A classic recipe in the South, lemon tea is one of those treats that is great year-round. This tangy, slightly bitter cocktail tastes great with any dinner.

2. Add water and ice until the pitcher is filled.
3. Let sit for 12 hours in a fridge.
4. Remove the allspice and cinnamon stick, and serve chilled.

The Pucker Delight

Are you a fan of the super tart taste of grapefruit? If you love sour and tart fruits, you're going to adore this pucker-inducing summer treat.

Ingredients:

- 1/3 lemon, sliced thinly
- 3 to 4 grapefruit slices
- 6 sour cherries, pitted and halved
- Honey (optional)
- Water and ice

How To Make It:

1. Use a spoon or a muddler to slightly squeeze the fruit. This helps loosen the flavors and allows them to diffuse everything a little easier.
2. Drop all the ingredients except the water and honey into the pitcher. Fill the rest of the pitcher with water and stir.
3. Let sit in a fridge for 1 day.
4. Remove the solids with a strainer, and serve.

Ingredients:

- 2 handfuls rose petals
- Ice and water

How To Make It:

1. Using a spoon or a muddling tool, muddle the rose petals until you start to really smell their fragrance.
2. Drop the rose petals in the pitcher, and add the water and ice.
3. Stir quickly, and place the pitcher in a fridge for 24 hours.
4. Serve, or use this water as a toner for your skin. Either way, it's great!

The Apple Pie

Something is oh, so American about eating apple pie with a little bit of cinnamon! This July 4th, enjoy a fruit water that has been modeled after this all-American treat.

Ingredients:

- 6 to 7 apple slices. (We prefer Granny Smith)
- ½ cinnamon stick
- ½ teaspoon allspice, wrapped in cheesecloth
- Ice and water

How To Make It:

1. Place the apple slices, cinnamon stick, and allspice in the bottom of the pitcher.

3. Fill up the rest of the pitcher with carbonated water and ice. Let it steep in your fridge for 12 hours.
4. Serve with a slice of lemon!

The Strawberry Smash Hit

This is one of the most popular fruit infusion water recipes in the history of fruit water. A classic cool flavored water drink if there ever was on, the Strawberry Smash Hit is a recipe that is sure to please even the pickiest water aficionado.

Ingredients:

- 5 strawberries, thinly sliced
- A handful of peppermint, thinly sliced
- ½ starfruit, thinly sliced
- Water and ice

How To Make It:

1. Muddle the peppermint, and drop it in the pitcher. Add the strawberry and starfruit.
2. Add water and ice until the pitcher is full. Let it steep in your refrigerator overnight.
3. Serve as is. It makes a great breakfast drink!

The Egyptian Classic

Pharaohs of ancient Egypt used to be very fond of rose water. In fact, their love of rose water extended beyond just using it for mere perfume – they drank it and used it in recipes too! Here's a quick recipe that nods to King Tut and Queen Cleopatra.

Ingredients:

- 1 handful mint
- ¼ cup diced pineapple
- ½ lemon, sliced thinly
- Water and ice

How To Make It:

1. Muddle the mint, and place it at the bottom of the pitcher. Add the pineapple and lemon.
2. Fill the pitcher with ice and water. Let it steep in the fridge overnight.
3. Remove the mint, pineapple, and lemon with a strainer. Serve chilled.

The Sugar-Sugar

Are you craving a sugary treat during the summer, but don't actually want to grab the sugary sodas on store shelves? We love this amazingly tasty summer treat.

Ingredients:

- ¼ cantaloupe, sliced very thinly
- 4 strawberries, sliced thinly
- ½ orange, sliced thinly
- Carbonated water, and ice

How To Make It:

1. Use a spoon to press down on all the fruits and berries to help loosen up the juices.
2. Drop all the sliced fruits and berries into the bottom of the pitcher.

1. Ever so slightly, use a spoon to smush the berries. You want there to be a little juice leaking out before you place them in the bottom of the pitcher.
2. Once you place the berries at the bottom of the pitcher, add water and ice.
3. Place in the fridge, and let steep overnight. Strain and serve.

The Chillo

Sometimes, you just want an infused water that is all refreshment, and that can also freshen breath. This is where this super cool, super minty infusion comes into play

Ingredients:

- 1 handful spearmint
- 1 handful peppermint
- Water and ice

How To Make It:

1. Muddle the two mint types in a bowl, and then place them at the bottom of a pitcher.
2. Add ice and water to the pitcher until it's filled. Stir.
3. Let steep in the fridge for 12 to 18 hours, and then serve.

The Mini Mojito

Mojitos are in. This is a less caloric, fruitier version of the popular bar drink. Viva mojito!

ingredients. Unlike the overly sugared lemonade you used to drink as a kid, this is a 100% sugar free option that will make your mama happy.

Ingredients:

- ½ orange, thinly sliced
- ½ lime, thinly sliced
- ½ lemon, thinly sliced
- Water and ice

How To Make It:

1. Drop all three citrus fruits into the pitcher, and fill the rest of it with water and ice.
2. Let it steep overnight.
3. If you want to, remove the citrus fruits and serve. Otherwise, just serve as is.

The Red, Light, And Blue

We named this one because of the fact that this fruit water has an incredibly light, refreshing flavor. You really can't go wrong with this one on July 4th.

Ingredients:

- ½ cup blueberries
- 5 strawberries, sliced
- ½ cup black berries
- Water and ice

How To Make It:

favorites have been used for centuries in beauty rituals. Now, they are being used to make a very refreshing fruit water blend.

Ingredients:

- 4 strawberries, sliced
- 1 handful of rose petals
- Ice and water
- A pinch of lavender (optional)

How To Make It:

1. Add the rose petals and lavender to the bottom of the pitcher.
2. Next, add the strawberries.
3. Fill the rest of the pitcher with water and ice. Let it steep in the fridge overnight.
4. Do not strain this fruit water. Instead, serve as is – ideally with chocolates of your choice.

Our Favorite Fruit Water Recipes For Summer

When summer is in full swing, nothing quite beats the heat like taking a sip of a super-refreshing fruit infused water blend. Here are our most refreshing blends in the book. All of these are best served very chilled, with lots of ice.

The Summer Stand

This recipe brings back memories of lemonade stands from your childhood with its deliciously tart

2. Fill the rest of the pitcher with water and ice. Let steep in a refrigerator for 12 hours.
3. Do not strain this fruit water. Serve as is.

The Ginger Mint Snap

Day spas are also known for their love of super foods…ginger being one of them. If you like to have your fruit water with a kick, try this one out.

Ingredients:

- 1 tablespoon of freshly sliced ginger root
- 1 handful of mint leaves
- Water and ice
- Honey (optional)

How To Make It:

1. Muddle the mint and ginger together. Drop them in the bottom of the pitcher.
2. Add water and ice to the pitcher, filling it completely. Let steep for 3 to 5 hours for a light flavor, and overnight for a stronger flavor.
3. Remove the herbs with a strainer, and add honey if you so choose. Serve chilled.

The Lover's Lane

Did you know that roses and strawberries actually belong to the same plant family? Both these day spa

- Water and ice

How To Make It:

1. Drop the lavender and lemon at the bottom of the pitcher.
2. Top with water and ice.
3. Let steep overnight, or for up to 24 hours, depending on how strong you want the flavor to be.
4. Remove the lavender-filled cheesecloth, and serve.

The Spa Lunch

Spa lunches always seem to have a balance of ingredients, and always manage to somehow just be *pretty*. This day spa inspired fruit water is a dedication to all those tasty lunches served at spas around the globe.

Ingredients:

- 1 handful mint
- ½ cucumber, sliced thinly
- 1 handful rose petals
- ½ cup strawberries, sliced
- Water and ice

How To Make It:

1. Muddle the mint. Drop the mint, rose petals, strawberries and cucumber into the bottom of a pitcher.

herbalists everywhere, we came up with this amazing infused water recipe.

Ingredients:

- ¼ cup mint
- ½ cucumber, sliced thinly
- 3 vanilla beans
- 2 teaspoons lavender, tied up in a cheesecloth
- Water and ice

How To Make It:

1. Muddle the mint, and add it to the bottom of a pitcher of water. Add the rest of the herbs.
2. Top the herbal pile with cucumber slices.
3. Add water to the filling point of your pitcher. Let it steep for at least 12 hours.
4. Remove the herbs with a strainer (and just pull out the lavender-filled cheesecloth), and serve.

Lemon-Lavender Water

We don't know what it is about day spas and lavender, but there's just something about these two that seem to go hand in hand. This recipe combines the rejuvenating flavor of lemon with a soothing flavor of lavender.

Ingredients:

- ½ lemon, sliced thinly
- 1 ½ teaspoons lavender, tied up in a cheesecloth

The Rejuvenator

Aromatherapy suggests that smells such as cilantro, mint, and orange can help awaken people who are feeling sluggish. We found out that it is the same with drinking essences of these same ingredients!

Ingredients:

- ½ orange, sliced and slightly crushed
- ½ lime, sliced and slightly crushed
- ¼ cup mint, cilantro, or basil. (Note: You can also try a combination of the three, or of any two you're particularly fond of).
- Water

How To Make It

1. Muddle the herbs that you chose in a small bowl. Once they have been sufficiently muddled, place them at the bottom of the pitcher.
2. Add the orange and lime.
3. Fill the remaining part of the pitcher with water, and let it steep overnight. Serve with a nice spa lunch.

The Herbalist

Many people who work at day spas swear by a favorite herb used in aromatherapy, or a favorite herb to add to spa meals. As a way to tip our hats to

- 1 small handful of rose petals
- 1 vanilla bean
- 1 pitcher of water

How to Make It:

1. First, you'll need to prep the majority of the ingredients. Muddle the rose petals and raspberries. Add the solids to the bottom of a pitcher.
2. Fill the pitcher with water. Cover it, and leave it to steep in the refrigerator overnight.
3. In the morning, use a fine sieve to fish out all the solid materials. Once you've done that, you're ready to serve it!

The Weight Loss Water

Cinnamon is a spa ingredient that is also known for being thermogenic, which means it's a natural fat burner. This super simple infused water can help you lose weight. Be careful, it can get pretty spicy!

Ingredients:

- 1 to 2 sticks cinnamon
- Water

How To Make It:

1. Drop the cinnamon stick into the bottom of the pitcher.
2. Add cold water, and let it steep for 1 to 2 days.
3. Sift out the cinnamon stick, and serve.

2. *Next, add the sliced and/or crushed fruit.* Once again, it's about helping the flavor get released here.
3. *Add water and ice (if you want to add ice).* Add enough liquid to make it to at least the ¾ mark.
4. *Let it sit for at least 12 hours if you want to have an intense flavor.* Otherwise, you can start drinking in as little as 3 hours. Believe it or not, it takes time for flavors to distribute themselves in water. Of course, the flavor distribution of the drink will reach a peak after about 18 to 24 hours. Fruit water, when placed in the fridge, can last up to 3 days. After that, it's time to make a new batch.

Day Spa Inspired Recipes

If you've ever experienced the true luxury that is a day spa, then you probably have been offered a glass of ice-cold fruit water while you wait for your masseuse. The following fruit water recipes are either day spa favorites, or inspired by day spas from around the world.

Red Dream Fruit Water

This fruit infused water has two ingredients often found in spa recipes – rose petals, and raspberries. Bon appetite!

Ingredients:

- 1 cup raspberries

you're looking for aesthetics, nothing beats a beautiful glass pitcher. Otherwise, anything will do.

- *Carbonated water, if you want a more soda-like fizz, is a good addition to any recipe.* Want a more soda-y feel to your fruit water? Just add carbonation!
- *A sharp knife and an egg slicer also can come in very handy.* Both are used for cutting fruits and herbs. The egg slicer just makes things a lot easier.
- *If you want to keep your fruits and herbs in the pitcher, we suggest adding a fine strainer to the top of your pitcher or jar.* This is totally optional, of course.

Once you have all this gear, you're ready to start making delicious fruit waters.

The Basic Gist Of Making Fruit Waters

Every fruit water recipe is pretty much the same, with minor details changed. If you haven't made fruit water before, you will need to know how to follow the basic pattern of making it. Here's what you need to do.

1. *Muddle the herbs (if necessary), and place them in the bottom of the pitcher.* This helps the herbs' juices spread into the water more easily.

that are infused in it. That's why many spas and weight loss programs suggest it for people detoxing from chemicals found in processed foods.

Making your own fruit infused water is easy enough to do, and a single batch can provide enough delicious taste for an entire day or two. All you need are the right tools, the right ingredients, and a little patience. What are you waiting for? Let's get started!

What You Need To Get Started

Making your own fruit infused water sounds pretty complicated, and it also sounds like the super expensive kind of project that you'd expect in very expensive restaurants. However, the fact of the matter is that making fruit water doesn't actually require much in terms of supplies. In fact, most of the supplies you'll need are dirt cheap, and probably already lying around your home. Here's a basic shopping list of tools you'll need. Many of them are optional.

- *You will need a muddler, a wooden spoon, or a mortar and pestle.* Crushing herbs and fruits before you add them to the water is a must in many recipes. We suggest getting a muddler, since its shape tends to make things easier with certain herbs.
- *You will also need a pitcher or a mason jar.* After all, you will need something to hold all the fruit infused water that you made. If

Every effort has been made to make this book as complete and as accurate as possible. However, there may be mistakes, both typographical and in content. Therefore, this text should be used only as a general guide and not as the ultimate source of information. The purpose of this book is to educate.

The author shall have neither liability nor responsibility to any person or entity with respect to any loss or damage caused, or alleged to have been caused, directly or indirectly, by the information contained in this book.

All rights reserved. No part of this publication may be reused, quoted from or reproduced by any means, including but not limited to printing, scanning, copying without prior written consent by the author.

Disclaimer and Terms of Use: This book is designed to provide condensed information. It is not intended to reprint all the information that is otherwise available, but instead to complement, amplify and supplement other texts. You are urged to read all the available material, learn as much as possible and tailor the information to your individual needs.

Made in the USA
Middletown, DE
18 June 2019